M000291355

www.TheKetoPrescription.com

The author, advisor, and publisher shall have neither liability nor responsibility to any person or entity with respect to any loss or damage caused or alleged to be caused directly or indirectly by the nutrition, exercise, and supplementation information contained in this book.

This book is not intended as a substitute for medical advice. Always consult a physician before beginning any nutrition, supplementation, and/or exercise program.

Information contained in this work has been obtained by the author from sources believed to be reliable and from personal experience. The author and publisher, for any information contained herein, assume no liability.

The topics addressed and the ideas expressed in this book are the subject of debate among nutritional researchers and professionals, and the authors are solely responsible for the contents of this book.

The Food and Drug Administration (FDA) has not evaluated the statements made about the supplements described throughout this book. The products described are not intended to diagnose, treat, cure or prevent any disease.

Book Layout ©2019 BookDesignTemplates.com
Book Editor: Qat Wanders (http://www.qatwanders.com/)

The Keto Prescription / Mel A. Ona, Jodi Nishida—1st ed.
ISBN-13: 978-0-9716585-4-7

Introduction

This is **not** your average keto diet book!

It's your "how-to" guide, your handy reference book, your working document.

This keto manual is designed to fit in your coat pocket or purse.

Our hope is that you write in it *extensively*!

We want it to accompany you to restaurants, parties, and, at least, the kitchen table.

We want to see food stains, oil stains, and dried-up cream cheese on the cover.

We pray it will contain your biggest dreams for your best health.

Who are we?

We are a **Gastroenterologist** and a **Doctor of Pharmacy**, who hope to <u>inspire positive change in healthcare</u>!

One of us is a mom, surfer, and entrepreneur.

The other is a singer/musician, writer, and actor.

We both **LOVE** dogs!

We both hope to improve your life in some way, shape, or form.

Come join us on this journey!

Doctor's Note

A well-formulated ketogenic diet, when mindfully applied, is a highly effective tool for "fixing" the obesity problem.

However, simply "cutting all carbs" and "eating all fat" is not advised nor effective in the long term.

This guide is primarily designed to be used in conjunction with a healthcare professional/provider who understands the ketogenic lifestyle and who is willing to support their patient in applying the keto lifestyle toward better health.

One crucial point to consider: the ketogenic lifestyle *may* be harmful **IF** a patient continues to take medications for diabetes and high blood pressure without modifying their medications as necessary.

For example, many patients have experienced dramatic improvements in blood sugar and blood pressure while following the ketogenic lifestyle. If they continue taking the same doses of medications for their diabetes and/or high blood pressure, then they may experience serious side effects (e.g. low blood sugar, low blood pressure).

We advise all patients to consult with their primary healthcare provider before embarking on a new dietary program—including this book/guide.

Our ultimate prescription is that you find and apply the nutrition program that supports your unique lifestyle and maintains your best health—for life.

The keto prescription may be the solution you've been searching for!

Let medicine be thy food and food be thy medicine.
-   **Hippocrates**

What Is the Ketogenic Lifestyle and Why Do It?

If you've been around since the 1950s, you know about living a low-fat life. This is approximately the time that our current US Dietary Guidelines were published.

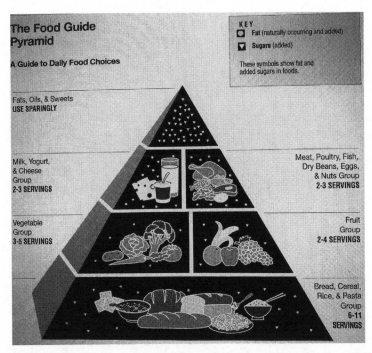

[Ref. https://www.cnpp.usda.gov/sites/default/files/archived_projects/FGPPamphlet.pdf, pages 2-3]

Where has this taken us as a nation?

Down!

We are sicker and more medicated than ever.

Why is this?

We started eating less fat and consuming more carbohydrates.

What are carbohydrates (or "carbs")? Carbs include breads, rice, pasta, potatoes, and sugars.

Where else are carbohydrates and sugars found? Fruit, soda, baked goods, desserts, dairy, and vegetables.

The average American consumes 200 grams of sugar per day.

The only math I'll ever ask you to remember for the rest of your life is this: four grams of carbohydrates turns into one teaspoon of sugar in your body.

200 grams = 50 teaspoons of sugar (FIFTY!)

You might as well grab a spoon, open the sugar container, and shovel 50 teaspoons down your throat. It's the exact same thing.

> ### Why is sugar bad for you?
>
> *Because it destroys our cells, muscles, arteries, gut lining, brain, skin, and everything else in our bodies through both inflammatory and hormonal/chemical pathways. Humans were not designed to run on sugar for fuel. Our ancestors thousands and millions of years ago were fueled by a different source: ketones.*

Fun fact: Babies are born in ketosis and remain in ketosis for as long as they're breastfed.

Ketones > Sugar (Glucose)

If you did your research and due diligence, you would learn that it wasn't until the agricultural revolution and invention of corn and grain-based oils that the American diet went south.

The acceptance and popularity of our low-fat guidelines were the invention of one man in the US: Ancel Keys. Mr. Keys was paid by the makers of Crisco oil to find a way to boost sales of vegetable oil over animal fat and lard. Very simply put, one man, one very poorly designed research study, and undereducated decision-makers in our government got our nation to where it is today.

The ketogenic lifestyle upends our US Dietary Guidelines.

It literally turns the pyramid upside down!

- Whole foods such as unprocessed meat/fish/eggs and healthy fats comprise the base of the pyramid.
- Non-starchy vegetables, nuts, and seeds fill the middle of the pyramid.
- Berries are at the tip of the pyramid.

KETO Food Pyramid

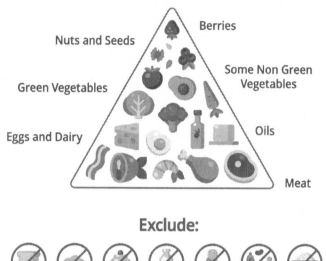

Nuts and Seeds

Berries

Green Vegetables

Some Non Green Vegetables

Eggs and Dairy

Oils

Meat

Exclude:

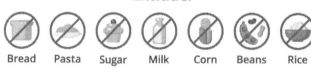

Bread Pasta Sugar Milk Corn Beans Rice

Keto = low carb, adequate protein, high healthful fats.

It is NOT fat that makes us sick. It's sugar.

Now before you go and do your "bacon happy dance," it's important to work with a healthcare professional who can put you on a well-formulated ketogenic diet designed for you.

Healthful fats are extremely important for our health, and, by eating low-fat for so long, we created numerous *new* health problems.

Fats and cholesterol are needed for healthy immune systems to aid in the formation of Vitamin D, which is important for bone health, the production of hormones like testosterone, estrogen, and progesterone, and forming healthy cell walls. These are just a few.

Looking at this list, you might be able to see connections to common conditions, such as autoimmune disorders, osteoporosis, infertility, low testosterone in men, etc. Fat is needed for life. Later in this book, we will show you lists of healthy fat food sources.

But first things first!

This book is an interactive guide along your keto journey.

First, we're going to get you to see what you eat, and then we'll transition to the ketogenic way of eating.

Fill out the following food/eating assessment:

Food/Eating Assessment

What I ate yesterday:

1.

2.

3.

4.

5.

6.

7.

What are my current beliefs about food?

1.

2.

3.

4.

5.

6.

7.

How To Get Started

Tracking Macros and Reading Labels

Getting started with the ketogenic lifestyle can be quite easy with the right guidance.

In essence, our goal is to switch from high-carb/high-protein/low-fat eating to a low-carb/adequate protein/high-healthful fats diet.

Carbohydrates, proteins, and fats are also known as "macronutrients." It is imperative to eat these in the right ketogenic ratios to induce the production of ketones in our bodies. Ketones are made from fats—both stored fat in our bodies and consumed fats from our diets. When we are in a state of "ketosis," we are essentially burning fat for fuel.

The best and easiest way to effectively monitor your macronutrient ratios is with a user-friendly app such as CarbManager.

CarbManager can be easily downloaded onto your phone or tablet and is free for the first 1-2 months. After downloading, set your macronutrient ratios as follows:

Total Carbohydrates - 5%, Proteins - 25%, Fats - 70% of daily intake.

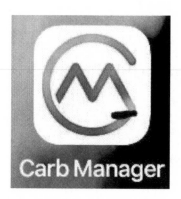

Once your ratios are set up, all you have to do is enter the food you eat daily, and it tracks your macros. With colored progress bars, you can see how you're doing throughout the day and adjust accordingly. Knowing where you are is extremely helpful because consuming too many carbs or protein will prevent you from achieving a state of ketosis.

Before getting started, it is extremely helpful to keep a food log for about one week.

This can help your healthcare provider assess your food choices and eating patterns in addition to your medical history. Some people can go cold turkey off of carbs/sugar, bear through a two-day bout of the "keto flu," and be fine. Others need to be weaned off carbs/sugar gradually and followed closely to manage side-effects and keto flu symptoms.

We will dive into this further in an upcoming chapter.

Nutrition Labels

<table>
<tr><td>

Nutrition Facts

Serving Size 2/3 cup (55g)
Servings Per Container About 8

Amount Per Serving

Calories 230 — Calories from Fat 72

	% Daily Value*
Total Fat 8g	12%
Saturated Fat 1g	5%
Trans Fat 0g	
Cholesterol 0mg	0%
Sodium 160mg	7%
Total Carbohydrate 37g	12%
Dietary Fiber 4g	16%
Sugars 1g	
Protein 3g	

Vitamin A	10%
Vitamin C	8%
Calcium	20%
Iron	45%

* Percent Daily Values are based on a 2,000 calorie diet.
Your daily value may be higher or lower depending on
your calorie needs.

	Calories:	2,000	2,500
Total Fat	Less than	65g	80g
Sat Fat	Less than	20g	25g
Cholesterol	Less than	300mg	300mg
Sodium	Less than	2,400mg	2,400mg
Total Carbohydrate		300g	375g
Dietary Fiber		25g	30g

</td><td>

Nutrition Facts

8 servings per container
Serving size   2/3 cup (55g)

Amount per serving
Calories   230

	% Daily Value*
Total Fat 8g	10%
Saturated Fat 1g	5%
Trans Fat 0g	
Cholesterol 0mg	0%
Sodium 160mg	7%
Total Carbohydrate 37g	13%
Dietary Fiber 4g	14%
Total Sugars 12g	
Includes 10g Added Sugars	20%
Protein 3g	

Vitamin D 2mcg	10%
Calcium 260mg	20%
Iron 8mg	45%
Potassium 235mg	6%

* The % Daily Value (DV) tells you how much a nutrient in
a serving of food contributes to a daily diet. 2,000 calories
a day is used for general nutrition advice.

</td></tr>
</table>

Lastly, learning how to read labels is of the utmost importance.

Notice that both foods contain 230 calories in the same serving size (⅔ cup). Both foods also are high in carbs (37 g).

However, one food (nutrition label on the right) contains more than *10 times* the total amount of sugar (12 grams versus 1 gram) per serving!

In fact, both foods contain the same amount of protein (3 g), carbohydrates (37g), and total fat (8 g) per serving.

Although both foods have equal calories and macronutrients (fat, carbs, protein), the food loaded with sugar may adversely affect your brain and body in the form of hunger cravings, energy dips, and inflammation.

Note: Total carbs (37g) minus fiber (4g) = net carbs (33 g net carbs)

Food Lists, Healthy Fats, and What to Throw Out

The best advice we can give on keto cooking and keto grocery shopping is this: don't overthink it!

It's natural for beginners to focus on carb sources instead of fats. But because healthy fats will comprise the majority of your daily caloric intake, it's important to know the options available. Here is a handy list. Do not run to the store and buy all of these. It's okay to slowly build your inventory.

KETO Food Pyramid

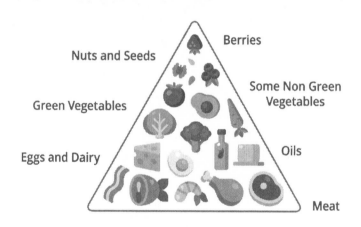

Nuts and Seeds

Berries

Green Vegetables

Some Non Green Vegetables

Eggs and Dairy

Oils

Meat

Exclude:

Bread   Pasta   Sugar   Milk   Corn   Beans   Rice

Healthful Fats

- Avocado/Guacamole
- Organic, grass-fed real butter
- Ghee
- EVOO (extra virgin olive oil)
- Coconut Oil
- MCT (Medium Chain Triglycerides) Oil
- Avocado Oil (including mayonnaise – we recommend the Primal Kitchen line)
- Walnuts
- Macadamia Nuts
- Pili Nuts
- Full-Fat White Cheeses (goat, feta, provolone, etc.)
- Cream Cheese
- Sour Cream
- Heavy Cream
- Hemp Seeds
- Chia Seeds
- Nut Butters
- 85% Dark Chocolate
- Canned Coconut Milk/Coconut Cream (for cooking)
- Unsweetened Almond Milk
- Whole Milk

Protein

- Fish (wild-caught preferred over farm-raised)
- Seafood
- Beef
- Chicken
- Pork
- Lamb
- Bacon
- Tofu
- Sausage
- Eggs

Carbohydrates

- Berries in smaller amounts
- Vegetables that grow above ground other than corn and peas

Artificial sweeteners

- Organic Stevia
- Monkfruit Sugar
- Swerve (for baking)

If you look closely at the general guidelines above, you immediately notice that A LOT of foods are included.

One of the best things about Keto is that this is the most satisfying, sustainable way of eating EVER.

In fact, knowing your options will allow you to do quite well on a ketogenic diet.

Foods to Avoid

- Salad Dressings that are not avocado oil-based
- Ketchup
- Mayonnaise that is not avocado oil-based
- Morton's Salt
- Vegetable Oil
- Canola Oil
- Sesame, Grapeseed, Sunflower Oil, etc. (anything that is not EVOO, coconut, or avocado oil)
- Sauces (e.g. BBQ sauce)
- Low-fat dairy products
- Cheese made in a factory, not from a cow
- Sugar
- Splenda, Equal, Sweet'N Low
- Sweets, candy, baked goods, desserts
- Food in a box (processed foods)
- Grains, oatmeal, etc.

Foods to Eat in Moderation

- Beans

- Legumes

- Soy-based foods

- Fruit

- Vegetables that grow underground (e.g. sweet potatoes)

Back to the saying "Don't overthink it."

Keto can be simple: a palm-sized portion of chicken or steak with steamed broccoli and a pour of melted butter.

Doctor's Reminder: the concept of Keto is simple (eliminate sugar and consume more healthful fats), but applying the lifestyle may require individualized guidance from a supportive health care provider.

Check out our website, www.theketoprescription.com, for programs and resources to help you follow and succeed with the ketogenic lifestyle. (Personalized coaching also available.)

Keto Flu, Managing Possible Side Effects, and
Vitamin/Mineral Supplementation

Did you know that sugar lights up more parts of the brain than cocaine and heroin combined?

Did you know that there are over 120 different names for sugar in our food?

It's no wonder that sugar is the single biggest addiction in our society. Upwards of 85% of our society is addicted to sugar, and they don't even know it. For this reason, when we eliminate carbs and sugar from our diets, we go through sugar withdrawal, a.k.a. "keto flu."

Keto flu can manifest differently in each of us, but the most common symptoms include: fatigue, weakness, lethargy, headache, muscle cramps, irritability, and dizziness. Basically, you feel like crap and feel like you have the flu. Picture a heroin addict going through withdrawals. This is you coming off sugar. Keto flu can last anywhere from two days to four weeks depending on how carb/sugar loaded you are.

Here are the phases to expect:

Keto Flu >> Keto Adaptation >> Ketosis >> Ongoing Adaptation

The symptoms of keto flu can be easily managed with the right coaching and guidance. All corrective actions include vitamins, minerals, electrolytes, and water.

Have these on hand:

✓ **Celtic Sea Salt or Himalayan Pink Salt**: Sea salt is an absolute must for anyone on keto. During the keto adaptation process, water can be drawn out of your cells, leading to headaches, constipation, muscle cramps, and weakness. By supplementing with sea salt, these side effects can be kept at bay. Don't be shy either. Sea salt is not harmful to our bodies, so you can generously salt your food, or add sea salt directly to your drinking water.

✓ **Green leafy vegetables**: 5-7 cups per day will give you the potassium and magnesium that you need.

✓ **Avocado**: Avocados are high in potassium, magnesium, and healthy fats. Be sure not to go overboard, though, as avocados also contain carbohydrates.

✓ **Hemp Seeds**: These tiny little seeds are unbelievable power-houses. Super high in magnesium and about 15 other vitamins and minerals, hemp seeds are an integral part of any well-for-mulated ketogenic diet. Sprinkle three tablespoons on almond yogurt for a super healthy keto snack.

✓ **Nori/Seaweed**: Seaweed is high in iodine and other minerals which help with keto adaptation.

Keeping your meals simple is the key to sustainability on keto.

Too often we complicate meals, and over time this leads to failed "diet plans."

Our advice to everyone has always been: Start with a palm-sized portion of protein, add greens, and add fat.

> *The easiest way to add healthful fats is a strategy called "sprinkle and drizzle."*
>
> *- Jodi Nishida, Pharm.D.*

Sprinkle chopped walnuts, hemp seeds, pecans, or macadamia nuts on your food.

Drizzle EVOO, coconut oil, avocado oil, or melted butter/ghee. You can even slice up some avocado or plop some guacamole on your plate. These are quick and easy fat hacks that will get you on the road to recovery in no time.

The incredible thing about keto is that once you're fat-adapted (when you've burned through your glycogen stores and burning fat as fuel), positive changes happen.

You'll immediately notice that you have fewer cravings, sweets are suddenly too sweet, you eat less, you feel full and satisfied, and you eat for nutrition versus habit or emotional reasons. These benefits are incredibly freeing for most people and liberate them from the prison of sugar addiction.

Sprinkle and Drizzle Fat Hacks

- EVOO 1 tbsp 14 g fat
- Coconut Oil 1 tbsp 13 g fat
- Avocado Oil 1 tbsp 14 g fat
- Kerrygold Organic Salted Butter 1 tbsp 11 g fat
- Ghee 1 tbsp 15 g fat
- Guacamole ½ cup 8 g fat, 4 g net carbs, 2 g protein
- Sliced Avocado, ½ fruit 10 g fat, 1 g net carbs, 1 g protein
- Chopped Walnuts ¼ cup 19 g fat, 2 g net carbs, 4 g protein
- Pecans, dry roasted ¼ cup 20 g fat, 1 g net carbs, 3 g protein
- Macadamia Nuts, roasted ¼ cup 21 g fat, 1 g net carbs, 2 g protein
- Hemp Seeds, raw, shelled 3 tbsp, 15 g fat, 10 g protein

Lunch or Dinner Options – 4 Easy Recipes

Pork and Brussels Sprouts Stir Fry

- 3 tbsp Avocado Oil
- ½ lb. boneless pork loin chops, cut into strips
- 1 lb. brussels sprouts, halved
- 1 stalk green onion, diced
- 2 cloves garlic, diced
- 1/3 cup low sodium soy sauce
- Hawaiian sea salt, Celtic sea salt, or Himalayan pink salt
- Pepper
- Optional: 1 tbsp granulated erythritol

- ✓ Heat 1 tbsp avocado oil in large nonstick pan over Med-high heat.
- ✓ Add pork and cook. Transfer to plate.
- ✓ Heat remaining avocado oil and brussels sprouts. Season to taste with Sea Salt and Pepper. Cook 6–8 minutes.
- ✓ Add garlic and green onion. Cook 1 minute.
- ✓ Add soy sauce, erythritol, and ¼ cup water—cook until sauce is slightly thickened.
- ✓ Return pork to pan and toss.
- ✓ Drizzle with EVOO, coconut oil, or melted butter.

Serves 4.
Per Serving: 6.25 g net carbs, 21.25 g protein, 15 g fat (depending on fat content of pork)
*Drizzle with healthy oils or butter and sprinkle with chopped walnuts for added fat and flavor.

Coconut Lime Drumsticks

- 3 cloves garlic, crushed
- 3 tbsp chopped ginger
- 1 cup chopped scallions
- 1 cup fresh cilantro
- ¼ tsp cayenne
- 1–2 tbsp granulated erythritol (optional) dissolved in ¼ cup chicken broth
- 1 cup canned coconut milk
- ⅓ cup lime juice
- 1 tsp grated lime zest
- 10 skin-on drumsticks

- ✓ In a blender, puree all ingredients except chicken.
- ✓ Cut 2 deep slits in each drumstick.
- ✓ Marinate in coconut mixture at least 1 hour.
- ✓ Preheat oven to 450 degrees.
- ✓ Lightly season chicken with sea salt and pepper and place on foil-lined baking sheet.
- ✓ Bake for 20 minutes. Flip over and bake another 10 min.

Serves 4.
Per serving: 5 g net carbs, 48 g protein, 23 g fat
* Drizzle or dip in healthy oils before each bite for added fat.

Orange Garlic Shrimp with Asparagus

- 14 oz large shrimp, peeled, and deveined
- 1 lb. fresh asparagus, chopped into 1 inch pieces
- 2 garlic cloves, minced
- 8 oz freshly-squeezed orange juice
- 2 tbsp avocado oil
- 1–2 pinches of sea salt

- ✓ In a large skillet, heat oil on medium-high heat and add garlic.
- ✓ Cook for 1 minute.
- ✓ Add shrimp and toss for 2 minutes.
- ✓ Add a pinch or two of sea salt.
- ✓ Add asparagus and fresh orange juice.
- ✓ Stir fry until shrimp are cooked through and asparagus are bright green.

Makes 4 servings.
Per serving w/o nuts or drizzle: 8.5 g net carbs, 28 g protein, 7 g fat
*This dish tastes amazing with both melted butter and chopped macadamia nuts or walnuts.

Cauliflower Nachos

- 1 head cauliflower
- ¾ cup EVOO
- Sea salt
- Paprika
- Garlic powder
- Cumin
- Chili powder
- Fresh parsley, minced
- 1 cup full fat cheddar cheese
- ½ lb. ground beef, 85% lean
- ½ packet taco mix
- ½ cup salsa
- ½ cup guacamole
- ½ cup sour cream
- Optional: jalapenos, olives

- ✓ Preheat oven to 425 degrees.
- ✓ Brown ground beef and add taco mix according to instructions. Set aside.
- ✓ Rinse and cut cauliflower into desired shapes.
- ✓ In a mixing bowl, add cauliflower, EVOO, 2 pinches of sea salt, and a couple sprinkles of paprika, garlic powder, cumin, and chili powder. Toss.
- ✓ Spread out on cookie sheet and bake for 20 minutes.
- ✓ Sprinkle cheddar cheese and bake till melted, about 5 minutes.
- ✓ Plate cauliflower and top with ground beef, salsa, guacamole, sour cream, and fresh parsley.

Serves 3.
Per Serving: 18 g net carbs, 46 g protein, 103 g healthy fats
*This recipe will help you meet your fat requirement for the day in one meal! *Fat bombs* are a convenient way to bump up your fat content for the day. They can also be used as a dessert substitute when the cravings kick in.

Strawberry Cream Cheese Fat Bombs

- ¾ cup full fat cream cheese
- 1 cup fresh strawberries or raspberries
- 4 tbsp salted butter
- 2 tbsp granulated erythritol
- 1 tsp vanilla extract

- ✓ Let first three items soften to room temperature.
- ✓ Puree strawberries in a small blender and add erythritol and vanilla.
- ✓ Combine all ingredients using a hand mixer until there are no clumps.
- ✓ Divide into ice cube tray or 18 round molds.
- ✓ Freeze for 2 hours.

Per round mold: 1 g net carbs, 0.7 g protein, 6 g fats

Tracking Progress (Measurements in inches)					
	Baseline	Week 4	Week 8	Week 12	Week 16
Neck					
R arm					
L arm					
Chest					
Abdomen					
Waist					
Hips					
R Thigh					
L Thigh					
R calf					
L calf					

Food Journal

Day: _____/Date: _____

	Protein (grams)	Carbs (grams)	Fat (grams)
Meal 1:			
Meal 2:			
Meal 3:			
Snack:			
Snack:			
TOTALS			

Laboratory/Blood Tests/Scan			
Date: __/__/__	__/__/__	__/__/__	__/__/__
Hemoglobin A1c			
Triglycerides			
HDL			
Fasting glucose			
Fasting insulin			
C-reactive protein			
apo-B			
LDL-P (particle number)			

FibroScan	CAP:	CAP:	CAP:	CAP:
	Grade:	Grade:	Grade:	Grade:
	kPa:	kPa:	kPa:	kPa:
	F: _____	F: _____	F: _____	F: _____

Journaling Pages - Identify YOUR "Why" for Better Health

I am committed to better health because:

1.

2.

3.

4.

5.

I must change my daily eating habits because:

1.

2.

3.

4.

5.

I must sustain a healthful lifestyle because:

1.

2.

3.

4.

5.

Eating Triggers:

1.

2.

3.

Keto Frustrations:

1.

2.

3.

Keto Flu Symptom Tracker:

1.

2.

3.

Symptom Tracker (energy, mental clarity, mood, sleep, digestion, skin):

1.

2.

3.

4.

5.

6.

7.

Body Transformation Progress

Date/Week #: _____

Body weight: _____

Body Fat%: _____

Fat Mass (Bwt x BF%): _____

Lean Body Mass: Body weight – Fat Mass _____

Total inches: _____

___

Date/Week #: _____

Body weight: _____

Body Fat%: _____

Fat Mass (Bwt x BF%): _____

Lean Body Mass: Body weight – Fat Mass _____

Total inches: _____

Body Transformation Progress

Date/Week #: _____

Body weight: _____

Body Fat%: _____

Fat Mass (Bwt x BF%): _____

Lean Body Mass: Body weight – Fat Mass _____

Total inches: _____

Date/Week #: _____

Body weight: _____

Body Fat%: _____

Fat Mass (Bwt x BF%): _____

Lean Body Mass: Body weight – Fat Mass _____

Total inches: _____

Ways to Kick Yourself Out of Ketosis

Burning through your body's glycogen stores and switching to a state of fat-burning is a huge accomplishment.

Ketosis, or using ketones for fuel not only has major health benefits at a cellular level, but also has tangible benefits all day long. When you are no longer a sugar-burner, you will feel like you're thriving.

The trick is to stay in ketosis as much as possible every single day. This chapter will cover the various ways you can kick yourself out of ketosis so you can avoid them and stay ahead of the game.

1. **Carbs and Sugar.** This should be obvious. Most of us can effectively stay in ketosis with the consumption of high healthy fats, moderate protein intake, and low carbohydrates/sugar intake.

2. **Artificial Sweeteners.** Many chemical sweeteners spike your insulin and have a high glycemic index. Read all ingredient lists and labels. Dextrin, maltodextrin, aspartame, saccharin, mannitol, and xylitol should all be avoided. Be cautious of pre-packaged foods and premade keto desserts. As a side note, decrease your consumption of keto desserts over time, and save them for special occasions. The goal is to wean yourself off sweets, and, if you do, you will notice your taste buds changing to a point where you no longer crave sweets at all. For most of us, this can be very liberating.

3. **Excess Protein.** One of the main reasons the Atkins diet fails is because it requires too much protein. Excess protein is converted to sugar (glucose) in our bodies through a process called *gluconeogenesis*. A general rule of thumb is to consume no more than a palm-sized portion of protein at lunch and dinner. The only time you might want to increase by ten grams protein per day is if your hair starts to fall out during the keto-adaptive phase. Don't worry too much about hunger. If you are consuming the right amount of healthy fats, true hunger should not be an issue.

4. **Frequent Meals.** Many of us can recall a time when we were told losing weight required eating four to six small meals throughout the day. This is wrong and can be damaging to our bodies for various reasons. If your four to six meals were not designed in a ketogenic ratio (5% carbs, 25% protein, 70% healthy fats), you were likely spiking your insulin levels each time. Insulin signals our bodies to store fat, whether it's your own insulin or exogenous insulin. Additionally, frequent meals can affect your gut microbiome over time. When we don't give our intestines time to rest between meals, detrimental changes occur. No internal organ system in our bodies should ever be overworked, the gut included.

5. **Stress.** Whether our stress is emotional, mental, physical or all of the above, it never does anything good for us outside of a true fight-or-flight scenario. Stress induces the release of cortisol, which in turn triggers an inflammatory cascade, causes our bodies to release sugar into our bloodstream, and increases cravings. This chain of events will kick you out of ketosis. Do your best to incorporate stress management techniques into your life, such as deep breathing, grounding, taking walks in nature, yoga, positive social interactions, and camaraderie.

6. **Excessive Caffeine.** Honestly, if you are in ketosis, you shouldn't require caffeine outside of your morning cup o' Joe. But it's important to know that by drinking caffeinated beverages throughout the day, you stimulate the release of the hormone adrenaline into your system, which then increases insulin secretion. As stated above, insulin stimulates fat storage (instead of fat burning), and this can kick you out of ketosis.

7. **Sleep Duration Quality.** Our sleep cycles are closely tied to our hormones and stress/recovery processes. Do your absolute best to get a good night's rest because a lack of rest affects our balance of hormones that regulate fat burning and fat storage, including adiponectin, ghrelin, insulin, leptin, and cortisol. If you have traditionally struggled with insomnia and/or tossing and turning throughout the night, get into ketosis! Ketones do wonders for sleep.

8. **Micronutrients.** Working with a keto-certified healthcare professional can make all the difference in the success of your ketogenic lifestyle. Too many people mistake keto for the "meat and cheese diet." Keto is not this. A well-formulated ketogenic diet incorporates food sources that supply adequate vitamins and minerals. Not only are they important for nutrition, they also help to keep keto side effects at bay during the early days when your body is building the machinery it needs to absorb and utilize ketones for fuel. Zinc, selenium, magnesium, sodium, and potassium are some micronutrients that are absent in the early days. Be sure to include grass-fed butter or ghee, sea salt, leafy greens, nori or seaweed, avocados, nut butters, and hemp seeds to your diet if you are aiming to get these through food.

9. **Estrogen-Mimicking Toxins.** Whether you do keto or not, we should all pay attention to these. BPA found in plastics, pesticides, certain chemicals in soaps, lotions, shampoos, and cosmetics can result in a host of detrimental effects on the body and should be avoided. These toxins also affect your fat-burning/fat-storage hormones and can kick you out of ketosis.

Eating Fat Does Not Make You Fat

We have been conditioned to fear fat. Yet, we'll throw hard liquor, beer, wine, cake, cookies, chips, donuts, hot dogs, soda, etc. down our throats like there's no tomorrow.

Picture the plumbing in your kitchen sink at home.

Now picture yourself pouring a bunch of bacon grease down the drain, adding some solid material, letting it cool and solidify, and there you have it! A clogged drain.

We believe that the exact same process happens in our arteries when we eat fat. This is fondly referred to in lipidology circles as "the over-simplification of fat."

> *People quit the ketogenic lifestyle for two main reasons:*
>
> ✓ *Their addiction to carbs and sugar takes over*
> ✓ *They believe that increasing their consumption of healthful fats will cause a heart attack.*

For your background knowledge and to help ease your mind, the content below comes from world renowned lipidologists. Lipidologists study fat, lipids, and cholesterol in our bodies. The *source* of the information that we implement in clinical practice is of utmost importance. None of the information here comes from anyone affiliated with the pharmaceutical, agricultural, or food industry.

Contained within the oversimplification model are the complete demonization of LDL (a.k.a. "the bad cholesterol") and the exalting of HDL (a.k.a. "the good cholesterol").

Unfortunately, it's not that simple.

Let's picture a typical scenario.

Your physician orders a fasting lipid panel or cholesterol test, receives the results, and makes medication decisions based on this snapshot in time. A chapter about all the details of your body's lipid system would be over 250 pages long. We don't have the space for that here, so we've included some basics that are intended to give you a better understanding of what goes on within.

Here are some definitions below.

Cholesterol (TC)

Cholesterol is a type of lipid, and there are many different types of cholesterol. It is a hugely important building block for survival. Cells can't make cell walls without it; it is an important ingredient in hormone formation (e.g. testosterone and estrogen); the human brain contains a whopping 25% of the body's cholesterol, and our immune system relies on it to function properly. These are just a handful of examples of what cholesterol is used for.

Every cell in the human body makes its own cholesterol. Cells do not get cholesterol from the food we eat. Every cell also knows how to get rid of extra cholesterol that it doesn't need. This intricate balancing act is called *cholesterol homeostasis*.

When your physician orders a total cholesterol test, the resulting number is the total of many types of cholesterol including VLDL, IDL, LDL, and HDL, to name a few. The value of your total cholesterol number is not as clear-cut as you think and doesn't represent a 1:1 ratio of the fat in your food. Physicians order lipid panels to measure your cardiovascular health and assess your risk of having a heart attack or stroke. The internal process of getting to the point of a heart attack or stroke takes many, many years and starts during childhood. This is a direct cry to watch what we are feeding our children in addition to watching what we ourselves eat as adults.

LDL (LDL-c)

LDL stands for low-density lipoprotein. Any time you see the word *lipoprotein*, think of a bus. Lipoproteins carry and transport cholesterol to different areas of the body. What is needed in that area gets dropped off, and excess gets picked up to be taken to the liver or intestines for elimination.

Unless you are getting an expensive, expanded lipid panel that measures LDL particle numbers, LDL traditionally is a *calculated* value. It's important to mention this because a patient with high triglyceride levels can throw off the accuracy of this calculation. High triglyceride levels are very common these days and can signify insulin resistance.

LDL has been dubbed "the bad cholesterol" for a multitude of reasons. Some are true, but many are false. LDL has many important functions, and one of these is to deliver cholesterol to body tissues and muscles from the intestines. Remember the bus analogy? It is an integral part of your lipid transportation system and is NOT a single, direct marker for cardiovascular health.

HDL

HDL stands for high-density lipoprotein. HDL is also an integral part of the lipid transportation system and has many functions such as picking up excess cholesterol from cells and transporting proteins. If we start to visualize the lipids and cholesterol in our bodies as components of a complex, organized, life-sustaining highway instead of artery clogging bad guys, we're halfway there.

HDL has been dubbed the "good cholesterol," but just because you have a high HDL does not mean you have excellent cardiovascular health. Again, there are many other markers to look at and factors to take into consideration before finalizing this judgment and putting patients on prescription medications.

Triglycerides (TG)

Triglycerides are simply the cholesterol particles within LDL that are transported to different areas of the body. Triglycerides tend to become elevated in people who eat high-carbohydrate/high-sugar diets. The Framingham Heart Study, which is the longest ongoing heart study in the US, showed that the combination of low HDL and high triglycerides is four times more predictive of a heart attack than a high LDL score alone.

To simplify this chapter and write it in a way that is easily understandable was quite the undertaking. The science of cholesterol and our lipid system is incredibly complex and difficult to understand with a few basic lab values. Here are some of the key take-home messages based on the very latest science:

1. Cholesterol is an important building block for our survival. Having too little leads to major deficiencies and functional problems.

2. Our brain and cells make their own cholesterol.

3. Standard lipid panels measure levels of total cholesterol, LDL-c, HDL, and triglycerides and are commonly used to make assessments of cardiovascular health or risk. A standard lipid panels measures the cholesterol in your plasma and leaves out the cholesterol in your blood cells, brain, and other cells in your body. It is NOT a complete picture.

4. Standard lipid panels look at a snapshot in time and is thought to only reflect the last three to four days of your life.

5. Our body has an intelligent, complex system called *the lipid transportation system*, of which LDL, HDL, and triglycerides are a *small* part. Until we throw it off with poor diet, this system is in perfect balance.

6. Lipid abnormalities begin during childhood.

7. Lipid imbalances can often be treated with diet. Increasing your intake of omega-3s, eliminating most carbs and sugar from your diet, and implementing intermittent fasting has been shown to have huge benefits.

8. The best indicators of cardiovascular risk to date are apoB and apoC3 test, LDL particle numbers, and lipoprotein(a) levels.

9. The problem with focusing solely on LDL is that we focus on fat intake and overlook the root cause of poor cardiovascular health: insulin resistance. Insulin resistance is caused by overloading our bodies with carbs and sugars.

Foods High in Omega-3s

- Mackerel
- Salmon
- Cod Liver Oil
- Herring
- Oysters
- Sardines
- Anchovies
- Caviar
- Flaxseeds
- Chia Seeds
- Walnuts
- Soybeans
- Brussels Sprouts (cooked)
- Hemp Seeds

About the Authors

Dr. Jodi Nishida's Journey

I want to warmly welcome every one of you to your new journey to achieving your best health.

Be excited!

I have embraced the ketogenic lifestyle since May 2017. I heard about "keto" from a friend. All she did was briefly mention it, and I went down a rabbit hole of research. Once I started, all these light bulbs started turning on in my brain. Little snippets of things I learned in pharmacy school came back alive. Keto concepts made complete sense, and I was fascinated with how backward modern healthcare obviously is! Five hundred hours of education later, I'm sitting here writing this book.

A couple of years ago, my father had a massive heart attack and almost died. Ironically, this major incident is also what healed our estranged relationship. While his physical heart was under duress, his emotional heart had finally healed. I felt it was my duty as his daughter, who was also a healthcare professional, to do a deep dive into what truly causes cardiovascular disease over time. My findings were so far from what's being preached in our guidelines that it was fuel for the fire.

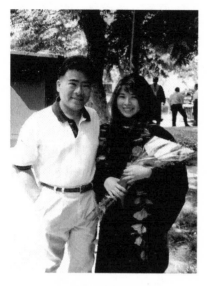 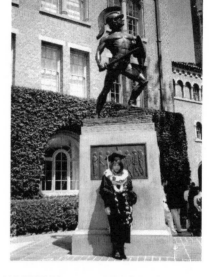

Jodi's father and Jodi, 1996   *1996 USC Pharmacy School Graduation*

Even though I'm a professional pharmacist, I am like many of you. My childhood was far from perfect and riddled with trauma, challenges, and hardship. At a young age, I learned to be independent, resilient, and self-reliant. My objective was to use my God-given intelligence to earn an advanced degree. This would provide me with a solid career and financial independence, living under no one's rules but my own. I was never the kind of person to take the straight and narrow path. I stood out like a sore thumb in pharmacy school. I almost got kicked out of high school twice for fighting on campus. I'm not a martyr either. But I'm really good at researching, formulating my own opinions, asking thoughtful questions, and bucking the system if needed. The bottom line is: I am not afraid.

We need people like myself and Dr. Ona to create awareness, lead change in healthcare, and upend the B.S. that has made us the sickest, most obese nation in the world. This singular fact should upset all of you. America has many things to be proud of, but not this. This is a disgrace.

It's important to outline my career because it tells the story of how I got here and how I know what I do. I am not your average pharmacist. Eight years were spent in both inpatient (hospital) and outpatient (retail) pharmacy practice. After going through some personal challenges and realizing I couldn't stand in a box all day counting pills, I left to pursue a career in the pharmaceutical industry. I was a newly single parent, and this difficult decision to work in the industry afforded me both time and money to raise my daughter. She was only three years old, and we needed to start over.

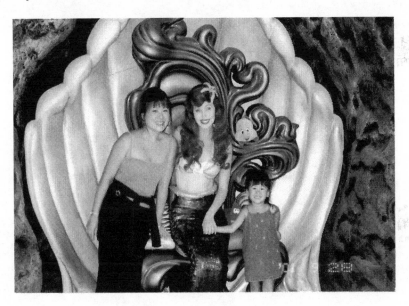

Jodi, "Ariel," and Kira 2001

I spent well over ten years in the industry observing, learning, and participating in the inner workings of medical sales. Although I didn't always agree with their methods, I can't say I regret any of it. Big Pharma invests hundreds of thousands of dollars in their sales people who are the "face" of the company to the client (physicians).

I learned how to manage a business.

I learned how to read people, relate to them, and speak with compassion and conviction.

I learned how to be an excellent listener and how to ask thoughtful, articulate questions.

Most importantly, I learned about myself.

My strengths and weaknesses were identified, explored, and worked through, and I truly walked away as a much better version of myself than when I first started. I met really nice people and scientists from all over the US and, for a small-town Hawaii girl, these interactions were invaluable. Had I stayed in a retail pharmacy answering phones, counting pills by fives, and pointing people to the "cough and cold" aisle, none of this would have happened.

Change can be good. No, change IS good.

When the time felt right, I left the pharmaceutical and biotech industry to pursue a career in pharmacogenomics. These tests take your DNA and map out which medications will/will not work for you. Think 23andMe on prescription steroids.

The information contained in those reports is invaluable to both doctors and patients in a world where physicians have minimal training in pharmacology, and do trial-and-error prescribing. Annual statistics show that more money is spent on managing side effects from medications than on medications themselves. That's a problem. Being directly involved in this field felt good, ethical, and useful. I collaborated with physicians across America, developed training programs and slide decks, was tasked with knowing all the new science emerging in this area, and helped doctors implement these tests into their practice. It was an awesome experience, which, unfortunately, over time, became an uphill battle.

On a political level, the pharmaceutical companies were really fighting this. It hurts their bottom line when physicians know ahead of time which medications to use and which to avoid. On a state level, insurance companies didn't understand the true utility of these tests and denied coverage. This is a common struggle with medical insurance companies. They often make decisions that don't make sense. When I saw clearly that this fight would be incredibly long and futile, I left genomics to go into the field of diagnostics.

There are few pharmacists who enter this arena. I now had this pillar of healthcare under my medical toolbelt as well. Diagnostics encompasses lab testing and rapid, portable tests which diagnose disease or monitor disease progress. It's truly fascinating to learn the technology in this field and witness it's application. In my new role, I worked closely with laboratories and hospitals, hearing their needs and frustrations with providing good, efficient patient care. They, too, struggled tremendously with budgets, medical companies, guidelines, restrictions, and conflicting interests. It was a valuable education.

My diverse professional background has truly given me a clear view of our fragmented healthcare system and who all the players are. It's important to understand that it won't get better for a very long time because of competing interests and the root of all evil: money.

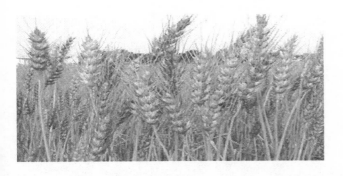

In 2015, Big Food made $390 billion on the following:

- Cereal
- Chips
- Candy
- Oatmeal
- Soda
- Ice cream
- Yogurt
- Cookies

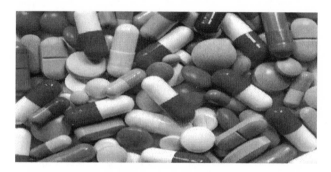

In 2016, Big Pharma made $383 billion on the following:
- Over-the-counter pain relief medications
- Oral diabetes medications
- Insulin
- Blood-pressure medications
- Cholesterol medications
- Blood thinners
- Heart failure medications
- Cancer medications
- Medications for erectile dysfunction

To be clear, I'm not sharing these statistics to slander anyone. What I'm hoping to do is provide transparency and empower each of you to take charge of your health. Instead of living and eating carelessly and then spending time and money on doctor visits and prescriptions, flip your script! This is avoidable! Do NOT rely on medications to fix years of bad habits. Start with what you're feeding your body every day.

Like you, I am also a patient.

In 2004, I was diagnosed with an autoimmune condition called *psoriatic arthritis*. It runs in my family, so I had accepted that I would suffer from this for the rest of my life.

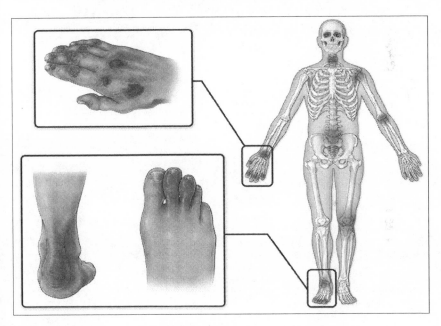

There were days when I would wake up and every joint in my body was inflamed, swollen, painful, and red hot. When it first started, my son was an infant, and there were days when I couldn't carry him because of my joint pain. These were very dark days for me. Like everyone else, I went to the doctor, had numerous labs run, and was eventually prescribed a medication. For 13 years, I injected myself in the abdomen twice a week to keep the symptoms at bay.

Back then, I ate a ton of rice, pasta, bread, and ice cream. I knew nothing about macronutrients and the benefits of being in ketosis. I relied

100% on my medication to feel better. I want all of you to know that sugar causes inflammation, and, since living the keto way, I have been off my injections AND pain-free/symptom-free for over 12 months. Because of my experience, I am now one of the most anti-medication pharmacists you'll ever meet. I am living proof that by tweaking our diet and going AGAINST our current dietary guidelines, medications are not necessary!

Having been living the keto lifestyle for 19 months, I don't go a day without it. I don't want to have to inject myself ever again. I've seen firsthand and through hundreds of patients that food truly is medicine or poison with NO grey area. Never in my life have I felt better from head to toe. I lost 15 pounds and two dress sizes, but this is barely the best thing about it.

Every night I sleep well.

Every day I have *clean*, sustained energy with no crashes.

I'm more focused and effective at work.

I can "mom" better.

I'm very even-keel emotionally. Even during my "shark week!"

My workouts are easier and recoveries are faster.

I FINALLY lost almost all of the post pregnancy pouch in my lower abdomen.

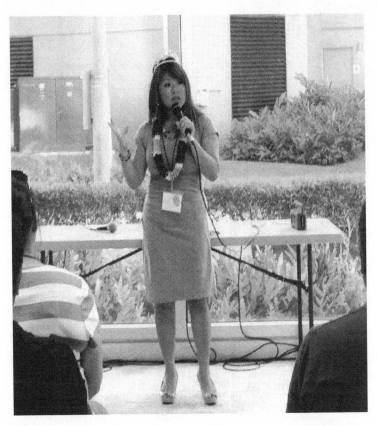

Jodi speaking at the first "Keto-Con" in Hawaii (a conference that she envisioned, planned, and produced)

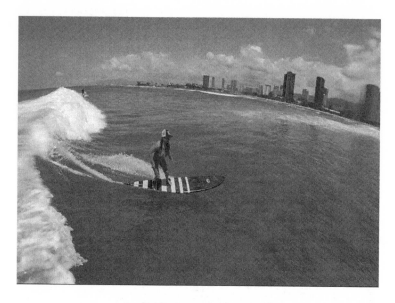

Jodi slicing up the surf!

I am clearer, brighter, healthier, and happier than I've ever been—all from eliminating carbs and sugar from my diet, increasing healthy fats, and doing my best to ensure that I'm in a state of ketosis as much as possible. Had I listened to the "guidelines" and Food Pyramid, none of this would be possible. Had I been too scared to buck the system, do my own research, and formulate my own medical opinion, I'd be in a very different place physically, mentally, and emotionally. I believe in the ketogenic lifestyle so much that I recently obtained my certification in low-carb, high-fat medicine. I'm committed to this medical field as much as I'm committed to all of you.

So... (deep breath)... welcome!

Please join my colleague, Dr. Mel Ona, and me on this amazing journey to achieve our nation's BEST HEALTH EVER.

Dive in, be open minded, ask thoughtful questions, and listen with your heart and intuition, and I promise you the journey will be just as great as the outcome.

Dr. Mel Ona's Journey

I had been overweight (actually *obese*) for much of my life and have weighed over 200 pounds at my heaviest.

Here's me (on the left) with my dad in 1996:

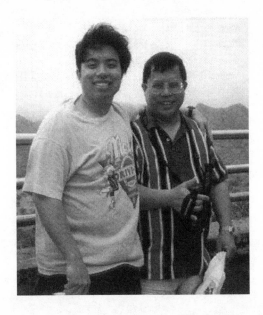

Yes, I was fat. And, of course, I tried every diet out there!

And you know what? I *succeeded* in losing weight on every one of those diets!

But, that's the challenge.

Haven't you started a diet and maybe even gotten excellent results at first?

But then, you deviated just a little bit. And then a little bit more.

Before you knew it, all the progress and results you achieved either stalled or reversed, and you gained all the weight back!

Well, that's exactly what happened to me EVERY SINGLE TIME.

I'd start a diet, stick with it for a while, but then I'd experience the death knell of all diets:

HUNGER!

So, I'd succumb to what my body and hormones were primed to do— eat!

And all the excess weight came right back.

In fact, here's a photo just one year (and three diets) later in 1997.

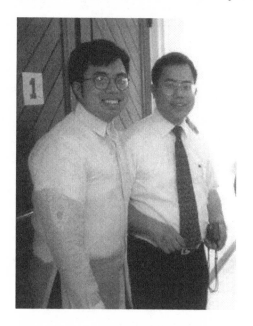

Mel in 1997 (left) with dad (right)

The photo was taken in the Philippines at my dad's inaugural opening of his free medical clinic for the underprivileged. I'm wearing traditional Filipino formal wear, which is a light dress shirt called a *barong*. I think the see-through material worked great in revealing my big belly.

I weighed approximately 183 lbs. at this time, feeling frustrated and utterly convinced that I would never get in shape.

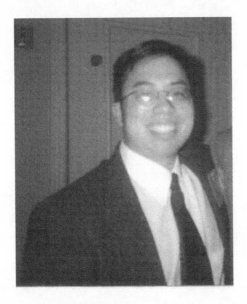

Mel in 1997 @ 183 lbs.

Actually, to give you an idea of what I was doing to "maintain" this unhealthy body weight, here is my typical diet from that time:

Meal One: Muffin or bagel with cream cheese

Meal Two: Large chicken parmesan sandwich, one slice Sicilian pizza, one can of regular soda, one dessert item (either a brownie or cookie)

Meal Three: Fast-food cheeseburger and fries or three to four large slices of pizza.

Water intake: minimal

Vegetable/Fruit intake: None or some shredded lettuce on the fast-food burger. Of course, I'd count the fries as a vegetable!

I'd continue to "snack" from dinner until bedtime on assorted goodies like chips or leftovers from previous meals.

So what exactly made me change my ways?

Pain!

Mental. Physical. Emotional. Pain!

I was *hurting* my health, and I was *hurting inside.*

I felt more and more disgusted with myself every time I tried a new diet and failed to keep the weight off.

My pain was *mental*—I felt frustrated and fed up.

My pain was physical—I felt tired and sluggish with daily activities.

My pain was emotional—I felt ashamed of my constant dieting failures.

But what got me mostly frustrated was how NUMB I became to that pain.
How often do we become so caught up in painful patterns and behaviors that it simply becomes part of our daily routine?

Well, that's exactly what happened to me.

That is, until I decided that I wouldn't settle for this poor fitness any longer.

It was another pain that finally prompted me to make a life-altering decision to stop eating junk and lying around and start eating nutritiously and exercising consistently.

I changed my focus from wallowing to a winning attitude.

I used the pain of feeling frustrated to feeling fed-up with my current state of poor health and fitness.

And that pain of NOT WANTING TO FEEL STUCK made me TAKE MASSIVE ACTION!

Massive action led me to experience massive results!

Mel's "Before" photo from May 1998

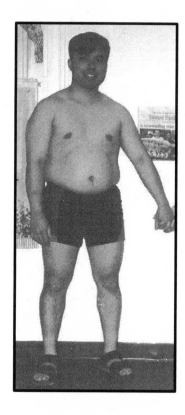

Bodyweight: 176 lbs.

Body Fat Percentage: 31%

Abdominal measurement: 40 inches

Body Mass Index (BMI): 30 (Obese category)

Mel's "After" photo from September 24, 1998

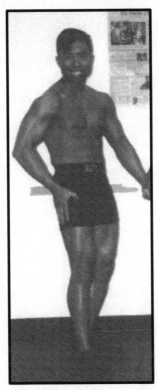

Bodyweight: 145 lbs.

Body Fat Percentage: 10%

Abdominal measurement: 30 inches

Body Mass Index (BMI): 25

In sixteen weeks, from May 24th to September 24th, I had developed a new, lean physique, and I was feeling on top of the world!

But let me be clear about one thing.
The journey was HARD.
It was NOT EASY for me to follow through EVERY DAY.
There were many times when I doubted my progress.
When I felt like giving up.
When my progress stalled.
When I slipped up on my diet plan.
When I cut back on my cardio intensity.
When I got "too busy" to prepare another meal.

But I pressed forward and focused on the next step of that journey...

- ✓ Cooking/preparing my meals...
- ✓ Packing my meals...
- ✓ Eating my meals...
- ✓ Keeping track...
- ✓ Exercising intensely...
- ✓ Getting enough rest/recovery...
- ✓ Following up with my coaches...
- ✓ Reading/reviewing my fitness goals...

...and getting absolutely CLEAR and FOCUSED on that "after photo"; it became a reality.

All of those actions required some measure of willpower, focus, energy, and time that I was COMMITTED to giving.

EVERY DAY!

And it was worth it.

Three months after I achieved the body of my dreams, my girlfriend and I broke up, and my healthy habits began to unwind.

When I felt down, I ate.

This changed my focus and made me feel different (note: I didn't feel *good*... just <u>different</u>).

The more I ate, the more I stopped thinking about our break-up.

The problem was that I ate crappy food—sugary, fatty foods.

Consequently, I slowly slipped back to my old habits (unhealthy eating and inactivity), and this caused me to gain back some of that lost fat weight.

It took only a *fraction* of time to destroy something that I had dedicated daily effort to build.

That's why "yo-yo" dieting is so common.

It's absolutely crucial to make a lifestyle change, and commit to eating right, exercising consistently, and supplementing intelligently on a DAILY basis once you transform your physique to remain healthy and lean.

So, here's my second "before" picture:

DAY: January 1, 1999

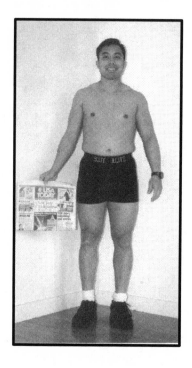

Bodyweight: 158 lbs

Body Fat Percentage: 14.5%

From the end of September 1998 to the beginning of 1999, I failed to follow through with the actions that had previously helped me get into the best shape of my life.

But then, a remarkable thing happened.

I got determined again!

I re-read those goals I had written down and re-ignited the passion for fitness within me!

I got back to following through with the healthful habits that I originally adhered to during my first 16-week physique transformation program.

And I succeeded in transforming my physique within a month!

DAY 28: January 28, 1999

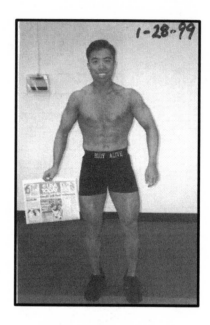

Bodyweight: 151 lbs.

Body Fat Percentage: 9.1.%

That's right, in only FOUR WEEKS, I was able to achieve a leaner and stronger physique than my original transformation, which originally had taken SIXTEEN WEEKS to achieve!

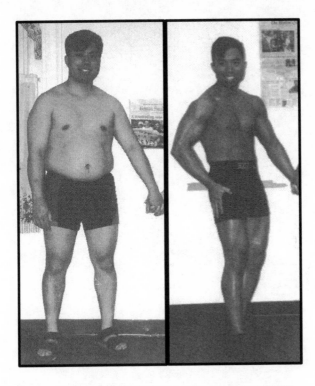

5/24/98	9/24/98
176 lbs.	145 lbs.
31% BF	10% BF
Waist: 40"	Waist: 30"

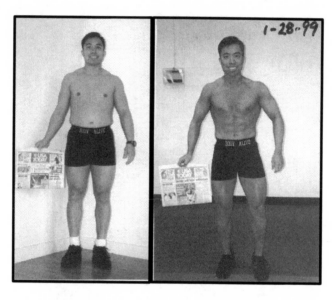

1/1/99	1/28/99
158 lbs.	151 lbs.
14.5% BF	9% BF
Waist: 31"	Waist: 29"

Body Un-Building (Medical School, Residency,

and Fellowships)

Are you struggling with your health?

Have you tried losing fat or changing your body for the better, only to find failure upon failure after trying multiple diets?

Have you succeeded in dieting, losing body fat, and perhaps transforming your physique for some time and ended up losing all of your progress, gaining all of your fat back, and feeling frustrated and more down than ever about your health and fitness?

You're not alone. I know exactly how you feel.

Remember when I mentioned that it took a fraction of the time to get back into shape after falling off the proverbial fitness wagon?

My story is not unique. I'm not special in any way when it comes to transforming your physique or becoming healthy once and for all. I was fat and out of shape for most of my life, but then, as a young adult in 1997, I was inspired by a physique transformation challenge made available by a supplement company in Colorado, and that contest galvanized my interest to pursue bodybuilding, fat loss, and physique transformation, and in 16 weeks, from May 24, 1998, to September 24,1998, I succeeded in transforming my physique from obese, with over 30% body fat, to lean, at 10% body fat.

I felt strong.
I felt confident.
I felt on top of the world.
Although I didn't win any challenges or contests at that time, I felt I had won a new life and a sense of confidence and certainty that I didn't have before.

But like yourself and many, many others, I became part of that statistic saying the majority of people who diet gain all their weight back and then some. From 1998 until now, I have experienced more frustrations and failures than fitness success.

In 2002, I achieved a remarkable transformation and competed in drug-free amateur bodybuilding. In fact, I attained a level of body fat that I had only dreamed about prior. In March 2002, I began another physique transformation journey, this time stepping on the bodybuilding stage and competing.

I lost a tremendous amount of body fat and competed with a single-digit body fat percentage in September 2002.

But...

My diet plan at the time was extreme, to say the least.

My total calories were 1,300 per day, very low carbohydrates, and very low fat, with moderately high to very high protein intake.

No doubt, this obviously worked!

However, after stopping the diet and eating normally again, from the time I finished bodybuilding in 2002 to the end of my medical training in 2017, I gained all of my previous fat back, added even more, and felt even worse.

I felt worse physically, I felt worse emotionally, and I even felt worse professionally. As a doctor, I couldn't maintain the healthy lifestyle I advised to my patients.

Overall, the reason why I gained back all the fat was physiological. Sure, some people might say I was lazy, complacent, and lacked willpower. For them, my weight gain all came from some character flaw.

However, I was just focused on more pressing and more important parts of my life at the time, such as getting through my medical training to become the best doctor I could be.

But whatever reason one may attribute to one's failures, the facts still remain that my body became adept at storing calories and body fat after a prolonged period of extreme restriction.

This is the reason why most people who diet succeed at first then stall out and gain it all back.

It's physiological.

So what was my solution this time around? I have tried so many diets, perhaps like you. And truly, I knew in my heart of hearts, and intellectually, that whatever diet I tried or did again would work, particularly in the beginning.

However, I was afraid that after those several weeks of being on that diet, the results would stall, that my mind and my motivation would wane, or my mindset deteriorate. I would feel as deprived and as crabby as I was before during those periods of extreme restriction, and I would end up blowing it all again. I thought all this until I met Dr. Jodi Nishida and seriously applied ketogenic principles to my daily life.

I was looking for a system, a plan, a lifestyle that could be sustainable. Sustainable in the sense that it would work WITH my physiology, not against it,

A lifestyle that enabled *fat loss*.

But I had questions.
Would I be hungry?
Would I feel deprived?

Would my energy levels fail to sustain me during busy workdays? The answer to all these questions was a resounding *"NO!"* with the ketogenic lifestyle.

I encourage you to visit our website, TheKetoPrescription.com, and learn about this particular way of losing body fat because it's not just working for me, but also for hundreds and thousands of others.

This is not a new diet.

It's not a fad diet.

It's been studied thoroughly by reputable scientific researchers such as Dr. Dom D'Agostino, Dr. Stephen Phinney, and Dr. Jeff Volek.

Go to the website: pubmed.gov and type in "ketogenic" and peruse the thousands of articles that have been published.

The ketogenic lifestyle is a tool. It's a choice. And it's one that I feel is worthy of analysis and application in your life, particularly if you have struggled with fat loss or health challenges such as diabetes and fatty liver disease.

It took TEN YEARS to not only undo the good health/fitness I built back in 1999, but also surpass the level of un-health that I previously experienced in 1996.

On August 1, 2017, I topped out at 201 lbs.

My body fat percent was in the obese category of over 30%.

I sported a 45-inch belly.

After I graduated in 2003—with a master's degree in nutrition no less—my health and fitness steadily unraveled.

From 2003 to the present, I ate my way through four years of medical school, three years of internal medicine residency, one year as an internal medicine faculty physician, three years of a gastroenterology fellowship, and one year of an advanced endoscopy fellowship that I completed in June 2017.

I got FATTER than I was nearly 10 years prior!

FACT: all the knowledge (medical, nutritional, gastroenterological—that's my future specialty) did absolutely NOTHING in regard to keeping me in shape.

Sure, I attempted "dieting" multiple times.

Rather than following the Hippocratic Oath, I was living a hypocritical one.
I struggled with my self-image and low self-esteem.

So what exactly happened?

How did I lose all the positive progress I had made?

Why did I let myself go and fail to stay in healthy shape?

Well, the short answer is that life happened.

I got so focused on other aspects of life—medical training—that I failed to tend to my own health and fitness.

You've heard the saying that hindsight is 20/20. Well, had I incorporated healthful habits throughout my 10-plus years of medical training, I'm certain I would have been in much better shape and felt more energy and vitality.

And that's why knowledge *isn't* power.

INTELLIGENTLY APPLIED KNOWLEDGE **IS** POWER!

But there's no use in wallowing in what could have or should have been.

It's better to understand how to make changes RIGHT NOW to get back on track and stay the course.

Throughout medical school (four years), internal medicine residency (three years), working as a teaching attending (one year), a gastroenterology fellowship (three years), and an advanced endoscopy fellowship (one year), I was under constant stress, lacked sleep, and chose to eat haphazardly and exercise sparingly.

That combination of stress, poor sleep hygiene, and a less-than-stellar diet/exercise plan simply led to my body creeping back to its prior obese state... and worse!

I had LOST lean body mass due to being older! (As we age, our muscle mass will diminish—a term called *sarcopenia*—unless we counteract that with resistance training/exercise and healthy living).

In fact, all that prior dieting and my past extreme caloric restriction essentially primed my body to go into preservation mode.

My hormones (those chemical substances that the body makes to regulate appetite and metabolic rates) automatically began to counteract what I was demanding my body to do.

While I was striving to lose body fat (albeit in a rather extreme way with drug-free bodybuilding), my body was under stress. When the body experiences stress, it will adapt.

Unfortunately, for many (extreme) dieters, the body will adapt by MAKING YOU HUNGRY.

Think of it as a thermostat.

When you set it at a certain temperature, the thermostat will sense the room temperature and then the heater (or air conditioner) will adjust accordingly.

Similarly, your body has several analogous thermostats.

Dr. Lee Kaplan from MGH/Harvard clearly explains the concept of the body's *set point*. (YouTube search: metabolic applied research strategy lee kaplan obesity.)

We have set points for blood pressure (some people have higher/lower blood pressure), hematocrit (some are higher, some are anemic), serum sodium levels, and, yes, even set points for FAT MASS.

My fat mass was set at a high level for much of my life. Our fat mass set point is influenced by a multitude of things, such as how we eat, our stress levels, our activities, our sleep quality (or lack thereof), and our genes.

I was able to change my fat mass with prior physique transformations; however, I never *permanently* changed my fat mass to a *lower* set point.

In fact, over the past several years, my body DEFENDED my original higher fat mass set point, and I got fat again!

What happened to me (and to so many others) is that I fought against physiology (feeling hungry and deprived) for a particular amount of time (many people achieve transformations in 12 weeks—I achieved my first transformation in 16 weeks and then six months to become extremely lean), and my body pushed back to get back to its original fat mass set point.

Once I succumbed to that raging hunger and stopped consistently exercising and resting/recuperating, my body's fat mass set point creeped back to its original state.

I use the word "creeped" because it's exactly like those garden weeds that you know are there, but you fail to tend to them, and, before you know it, you have a weed garden!

The physiology of my fat mass set point was inappropriately set too high.

Several things can lower your fat mass set point:

- Lifestyle modifications: diet (not restrictions per se, but changing the composition of what one eats), exercise, sleep hygiene, bio-rhythm optimization
- Medications
- Surgery

Different people will respond to different strategies to lower the set point.

My permanent transformation now involves a major mindset reset.

Rather than fighting my body's physiology, I am focusing on living in a way that encourages my body to be at a lower fat mass set point.

Not by restrictive measures.

Not by forcing my body to drastically lose fat.

Not by doing anything extreme.

To do this, first and foremost, I changed my mindset.

Then I focused on reducing stress.

I changed my sleep quality for the better.

So far, the body fat is coming off rather imperceptibly and without me feeling deprived.

The ketogenic lifestyle is one effective way to "reset" the fat mass set point to healthier levels without feeling raging hunger pangs, mental misery, or deprivation.

REMINDER:

Don't just settle for maintaining. Instead, keep setting new goals, and continue striving for daily improvement.

If you slip up, just refocus and recharge your commitment to excellence!

NOTE THE TREND...

Mel in 1997

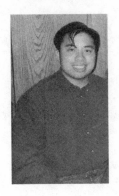

Mel in 1998

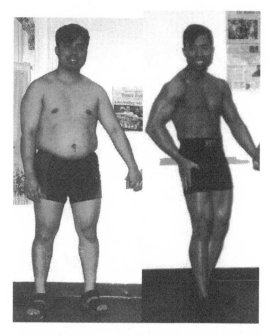

May 24, 1998   September 24, 1998

Mel in 1999

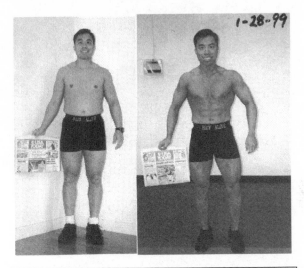

| 1/1/99 (Day 1) | 1/28/99 (Day 28) |

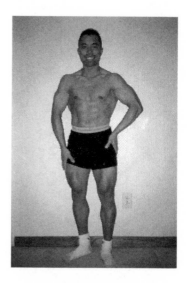

April 2001

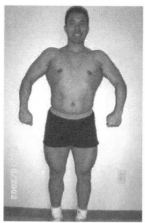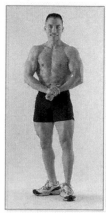

March 2002   **August 2002**

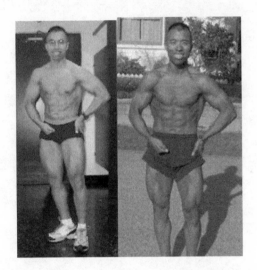

Bodybuilder lean (September 2002)

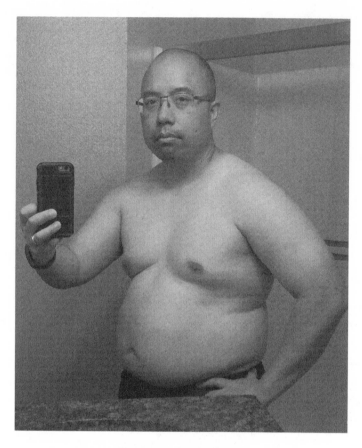

Fat regain (2017)

Yo-Yo Dieting... No, No!

If you were to look at my numbers (body weight especially), you may think that this trend is the typical "yo-yo" diet syndrome.

My bodyweight "numbers":
1997: 183 lbs.
1998: 176 lbs.; 145 lbs.
1999: 158 lbs.; 151 lbs.
2001: 148 lbs.; 155 lbs.
2002: 160 lbs.; 140 lbs.

Weight loss, weight gain, weight loss, weight gain.

A very typical yo-yo pattern.

HOWEVER, if you look more closely, you'll notice that with each subsequent weight GAIN, I built MORE lean body mass rather than fat mass.

In other words, over time, I was getting LEANER! Most "yo-yo" dieters get FATTER, lose muscle, and become unhealthier over time.

My percentage body fat "numbers":
1997: 33% body fat
1998: 31% body fat; 10% body fat
1999: 14.5% body fat; 9% body fat
2001: 7.5% body fat; 8.5% body fat
2002: 17% body fat; 5.0% body fat

Again, the weight loss was fat and the weight regain was mostly lean body mass.

My body numbers from the beginning of medical school until 2017:

2005 (started medical school): 160 lbs.

2009 (started internal medicine residency): 175 lbs.
2013 (started gastroenterology fellowship): 185 lbs.
2015 (mid-way through final year of GI fellowship): 200 lbs.
May 10, 2016 (age 45): 175 lbs.
August 1, 2017 (age 46, after completion of advanced endoscopy fellowship): 201 lbs.

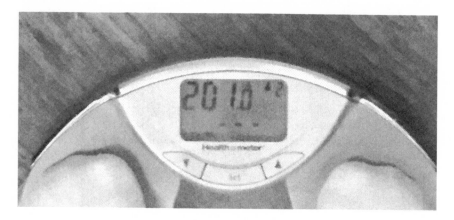

August 2017: 201 lbs

My body weight got all the way back (and more) to the highest it ever was.

And I LOST lean body mass!

How did this happen?!

After all, I'm a DOCTOR! I'm board-certified in internal medicine! Plus, I have a master's degree in nutritional biochemistry and metabolism!

Aren't I supposed to be an expert in health?

My body and physiology got back to my fat mass set point, with the gradual weight gain driven by appetite hormones causing me to eat more.

I don't blame my genetics, but I do have a *tendency* toward weight gain.

This tendency PLUS an *obesogenic environment* resulted in the excess body fat I gained steadily over the years.

What is an **obesogenic** *environment?*

- *Lots of stress (the disruptive/bad kind...I wasn't exercising much at the time of weight regain)*
- *Low quality sleep*
- *Disrupted biorhythms*
- *Insulin-spiking meals (processed foods, refined carbohydrates)*
- *Lack of exercise*
- *Lack of healthy muscle (from lack of exercise)*

What can reset a fat mass set point to healthier levels?

- Eating whole food that's unprocessed and unrefined
- Improving sleep hygiene (better quality consistent sleep)
- Consistent exercise to build healthy muscle
- Mental conditioning
- Associating with positive, fitness-minded people
- Staying accountable to health coaches

This brings us to the present day.

I've completed my medical training.

My new career is over one year old (time flies!), and I've joined a thriving gastroenterology private practice.

Fitness-wise, I'm making progress every day.

I invite you to follow along on this fitness journey with me and Dr. Jodi Nishida.

After countless missteps and failures, I'm finally back on track!

I've written thousands of medical prescriptions for patients.

Now, Dr. Nishida and I are prescribing the ketogenic lifestyle for those who are committed to lifelong health and vitality.

Check out the following timeline of my transformation throughout the stages of my graduate/medical training on the next page. (By the way, I'm still and always will be a "work-in-progress," as there's always something we can improve/enhance/learn/apply in our lives!)

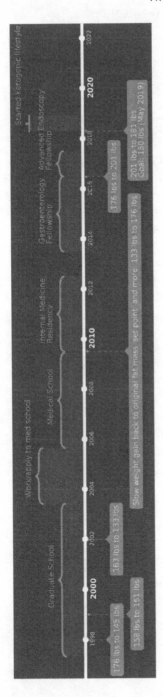

Recommended Keto Resources

- **Ken D. Berry, MD** (Instagram and YouTube: KenDBerryMD): Dr. Berry is a board-certified family physician who has treated over 20,000 unique patients during his career spanning over a decade. He explains how you can use diet and lifestyle to stay healthy and happy. He has over 300,000 subscribers and over 13 million views of his videos about the ketogenic diet, intermittent fasting, thyroid health, hormone optimization, and much more. He's the bestselling author of the controversial book, *Lies My Doctor Told Me.*

- **Dom D'Agostino, PhD** (www.ketonutrition.org): Dr. D'Agostino is a highly-respected and sought-after expert on nutritional science. He is a tenured associate professor at the University of South Florida and teaches at the Morsani College of Medicine in the Department of Molecular Pharmacology and Physiology. His research focuses on neuropharmacology, medical biochemistry, physiology, and neuroscience. He is also a research scientist at the Institute for Human and Machine Cognition studying how to optimize the safety, health, and resilience of warfighters and astronauts. (More information about Dr. D'Agostino: https://www.ketonutrition.org/about/)

- **Peter Attia, MD** (https://peterattiamd.com/category/ketosis/): This explores Dr. Peter Attia's comprehensive, in-depth personal journey with ketosis.

- **Virta Health** (www.virtahealth.com): Virta Health is a company focused on diabetes reversal founded by renowned research scientists/academicians Dr. Stephen Phinney and Dr. Jeff Volek.

- **John Limansky, MD** (www.johnlimanskymd.com): Dr. John Limansky is "The Keto Doctor" and a board-certified physician in internal medicine).

- **Ryan Lowery, Ph.D.** (www.ketogenic.com): Dr. Ryan Lowery is committed to supporting, inspiring, and educating people on the benefits of living a ketogenic lifestyle. He is the author of *The Ketogenic Bible: The Authoritative Guide to Ketosis.*

- **Nina Teicholz** (www.ninateicholz.com): Nina Teicholz is a *New York Times* bestselling author of the groundbreaking book, *The Big Fat Surprise*, which was named a Top Science Book of 2014 by *The Economist*. She is the founder/Executive Director of The Nutrition Coalition (non-partisan, non-profit with no industry ties).

Made in the USA
San Bernardino, CA
30 August 2019